The Natural Vision Healer:

A Doctor's Guide to Curing Myopia without Glasses or Surgery

Dr. James P. West

Table of Contents

Chapter 1. Introduction

(Nancy) - This book has been a game changer for me! As a long-time sufferer of myopia, I had resigned myself to a life of dependence on glasses and contacts. However, after purchasing and reading 'The Natural Vision Healer' by Dr. James P. West on Amazon bookstore , I discovered simple and effective techniques for improving my eyesight that I could easily integrate into my daily routine.

Not only did the exercises and lifestyle tips outlined in the book help me to gradually reduce my reliance on corrective lenses, but I also gained a deeper understanding of the root causes of myopia and how to maintain good eye health. The clear and concise explanations and step-by-step guidance made it easy for me to follow along and see real results.

I highly recommend this book to anyone looking to improve their eyesight and take control of their eye health. Whether you have mild myopia or severe nearsightedness, this doctor-written guide offers a natural and holistic approach to improving your vision."

Overview of Myopia

Myopia, also known as nearsightedness, is a common refractive error of the eye that affects millions of people worldwide. It occurs when the eye is too long or the cornea is too curved, causing light to focus in front of the retina instead of directly on it. This results in the ability to see objects up close clearly, but distant objects appear blurry.

Myopia is a growing concern in many countries, as the prevalence of the condition has increased significantly in recent years. This is partly due to increased screen time and a lack of outdoor light exposure, as well as genetics and environmental factors.

While glasses and contacts can correct the symptoms of myopia, they do not address the underlying causes of the condition. In some cases, myopia can progress to a more serious form known as high myopia, which can increase the risk of eye diseases and vision loss.

The good news is that there is growing evidence that myopia can be prevented or even reversed through simple and effective lifestyle changes and vision improvement techniques. In this book, we will explore the root causes of myopia and provide a comprehensive guide to improving your vision naturally.

Understanding the Causes and Consequences of Nearsightedness

Myopia is a complex condition that can have multiple causes, including genetics, environmental factors, and visual habits. Some of the most common contributing factors include:

Extended screen time: Spending prolonged periods of time looking at screens can cause eye strain and increase the risk of myopia.

Lack of outdoor light exposure: Exposure to natural light is important for maintaining good eye health, as it helps regulate the production of the hormone melatonin, which has been linked to myopia.

Close-up work: Engaging in close-up activities such as reading, writing, and using a computer can increase the risk of myopia, especially if they are done for extended periods of time.

Family history: Myopia tends to run in families, indicating a strong genetic component.

In addition to these causes, other factors such as stress, diet, and lifestyle habits can also play a role in the development of myopia.

If left untreated, myopia can have serious consequences for vision and eye health. It can lead to an increased risk of eye diseases such as glaucoma, cataracts, and retinal detachment, as well as decreased quality of life due to reduced visual acuity. High myopia, which is a more severe form of the condition, can even result in blindness.

By understanding the causes and consequences of myopia, you can take steps to reduce your risk and improve your eye health. In this book, we will explore the latest research on the subject and provide practical tips and techniques for improving your vision and reducing your risk of myopia.

A Holistic Approach to Improving Vision

Traditional approaches to treating myopia often rely on corrective lenses or surgery to correct the symptoms, but they do not address the underlying causes of the condition. In this book, we take a holistic approach to improving vision by addressing not only the physical aspects of myopia, but also the mental, emotional, and lifestyle factors that contribute to it.

Our approach is based on the idea that the health of the eyes and the visual system is interrelated with the overall health of the body and mind. By taking care of your overall well-being and adopting healthy habits, you can improve your eye health and reduce your risk of myopia.

In this book, we will explore the latest research on the subject and provide practical tips and techniques for improving your vision and reducing your risk of myopia, including:

Lifestyle changes such as reducing screen time, eating a healthy diet, and getting regular exercise

Vision improvement techniques such as palming, sunning, eye massages, and dynamic visual training

Customizing your vision improvement plan by setting realistic goals and monitoring your progress

Maintaining good eye health through regular eye exams, protecting your eyes from harm, and continuing your vision improvement journey

Our holistic approach to improving vision is based on the latest scientific research and incorporates proven techniques for improving eye health and reducing the risk of myopia. Whether you have mild myopia or severe nearsightedness, this book offers a natural and effective solution for improving your vision and maintaining good eye health.

Chapter 2. Lifestyle Changes for Better Eye Health

Lifestyle changes are an important part of improving eye health and reducing the risk of myopia. In this book, we will explore the latest research on the subject and provide practical tips and techniques for making changes that can have a positive impact on your vision. Some of the lifestyle changes we will discuss include:

Reducing screen time: Spending prolonged periods of time looking at screens can cause eye strain and increase the risk of myopia. We will provide tips for reducing screen time and minimizing eye strain, including taking frequent breaks and using blue light filters.

Getting outside: Spending time in natural light is important for maintaining good eye health and reducing the risk of myopia. We will discuss the benefits of spending time outdoors, as well as practical tips for incorporating more outdoor activities into your daily routine.

Eating a healthy diet: Eating a diet rich in nutrients and antioxidants can support eye health and reduce the risk of myopia. We will provide recommendations for foods that are beneficial for the eyes, as well as tips for a healthy and balanced diet.

Getting regular exercise: Exercise has been shown to improve eye health and reduce the risk of myopia. We will discuss the benefits of physical activity, as well as tips for incorporating exercise into your daily routine.

By incorporating these lifestyle changes into your daily routine, you can improve your eye health and reduce your risk of myopia. In this book, we will provide guidance and support to help you make these changes and achieve your vision improvement goals.

The Importance of Outdoor Light Exposure

Outdoor light exposure is an important factor in maintaining good eye health and reducing the risk of myopia. In this book, we will discuss the latest research on the subject and provide practical tips and techniques for maximizing the benefits of outdoor light exposure.

Exposure to natural light is important for regulating the production of the hormone melatonin, which has been linked to myopia. Additionally, outdoor light exposure helps the eyes to focus and track objects, which can improve visual acuity and reduce the risk of myopia.

However, many people spend a significant amount of time indoors, which can lead to decreased light exposure and an increased risk of myopia. In this book, we will provide tips for maximizing your outdoor light exposure, including spending time outdoors, using natural light in your home, and taking breaks from screens.

We will also discuss the benefits of sunning, which is a technique for exposing the eyes to natural light and improving eye health. Sunning involves looking at the sun for a few minutes each day, while taking precautions to protect your eyes from harmful UV rays.

By incorporating outdoor light exposure into your daily routine, you can improve your eye health and reduce your risk of myopia. Whether you are spending time in natural light or using sunning techniques, we will provide guidance and support to help you make the most of your outdoor light exposure.

Eating for Eye Health

Diet plays an important role in maintaining good eye health and reducing the risk of myopia. In this book, we will discuss the latest research on the subject and provide practical tips and techniques for eating a healthy and balanced diet that supports eye health.

Eating a diet rich in nutrients and antioxidants can help to protect the eyes from damage and reduce the risk of myopia. Some of the key nutrients and foods that are beneficial for the eyes include:

Vitamin A: found in foods such as carrots, sweet potatoes, and spinach

Vitamin C: found in foods such as citrus fruits, bell peppers, and broccoli

Omega-3 fatty acids: found in foods such as fatty fish, chia seeds, and flaxseeds

Zinc: found in foods such as oysters, pumpkin seeds, and beef

In addition to eating a healthy and balanced diet, we will also discuss the importance of avoiding processed foods, sugary drinks, and excessive caffeine, which can have a negative impact on eye health.

By incorporating eye-friendly foods into your diet and avoiding those that can be harmful, you can improve your eye health and reduce your risk of myopia. In this book, we will provide guidance and support to help you make healthy food choices and achieve your vision improvement goals.

Minimizing Screen Time and Digital Eye Strain

Spending prolonged periods of time looking at screens can cause eye strain and increase the risk of myopia. In this book, we will discuss the latest research on the subject and provide practical tips and techniques for minimizing screen time and reducing digital eye strain.

Digital eye strain is a common problem that is caused by the prolonged use of electronic devices, such as smartphones, laptops, and televisions. Symptoms of digital eye strain can include eye fatigue, headache, and blurred vision.

To reduce the risk of digital eye strain and myopia, it is important to minimize screen time and take frequent breaks from screens. In this book, we will provide tips for reducing screen time, including setting limits on device usage, taking breaks every 20 minutes, and using blue light filters.

We will also discuss the benefits of using proper lighting when working with screens, and provide tips for reducing glare and reflections. Additionally, we will discuss the importance of using good posture when using electronic devices, which can help to reduce eye strain and prevent myopia.

By minimizing screen time and reducing digital eye strain, you can improve your eye health and reduce your risk of myopia. In this book, we will provide guidance and support to help you make these changes and achieve your vision improvement goals.

Reducing Stress and Relaxing the Eyes

Stress and tension can have a negative impact on eye health and increase the risk of myopia. In this book, we will discuss the latest research on the subject and provide practical tips and techniques for reducing stress and relaxing the eyes.

Stress can cause the eyes to tense up, leading to eye strain and fatigue. Additionally, stress can interfere with the body's ability to regulate hormones and maintain good eye health.

To reduce stress and relax the eyes, it is important to engage in stress-reducing activities, such as meditation, yoga, and deep breathing exercises. In this book, we will provide tips for reducing stress, including setting aside time for relaxation, practicing mindfulness, and engaging in physical activity.

We will also discuss the benefits of eye relaxation exercises, which can help to reduce eye strain and improve eye health. These exercises can include techniques such as palming, eye movements, and using vision therapy techniques.

By reducing stress and relaxing the eyes, you can improve your eye health and reduce your risk of myopia. In this book, we will provide guidance and support to help you make these changes and achieve your vision improvement goals.

Chapter 3. Vision Improvement Techniques

There are a number of techniques and exercises that can be used to improve vision and reduce the risk of myopia. In this book, we will discuss the latest research on the subject and provide practical tips and techniques for improving vision.

Some of the vision improvement techniques that we will cover include:

Vision Therapy Exercises: These exercises can help to strengthen the eye muscles and improve visual acuity. They can include techniques such as eye tracking, focusing exercises, and binocular vision exercises.

Light Therapy: Light therapy can help to regulate the circadian rhythm and improve visual acuity. This can include techniques such as sun gazing, spending time in bright light, and using light therapy lamps.

Visualization Techniques: Visualization techniques can help to improve visual acuity and reduce eye strain. These techniques can include imagining bright and clear images, and visualizing a peaceful and relaxing environment.

Palming: Palming is a technique that involves covering the eyes with the palms of the hands to reduce eye strain and improve eye health.

By incorporating these techniques and exercises into your daily routine, you can improve your vision and reduce your risk of myopia. In this book, we will provide guidance and support to help you implement these techniques and achieve your vision improvement goals.

Palming and Sunning

Palming and sunning are two techniques that can be used to improve vision and reduce the risk of myopia. In this book, we will discuss the latest research on the subject and provide practical tips and techniques for incorporating these techniques into your daily routine.

Palming is a technique that involves covering the eyes with the palms of the hands to reduce eye strain and improve eye health. This technique works by blocking out light and allowing the eyes to rest and relax. It is best practiced in a quiet and dark environment, and can be performed several times a day.

Sunning is a technique that involves exposing the eyes to bright light, such as sunlight. This technique can help to regulate the circadian rhythm, improve visual acuity, and reduce the risk of myopia. Sunning is best performed in the morning, when the sun is at its brightest. It is recommended to start with short periods of sun exposure and gradually increase the amount of time spent sunning.

By incorporating palming and sunning into your daily routine, you can improve your vision and reduce your risk of myopia. In this book, we will provide guidance and support to help you implement these techniques and achieve your vision improvement goals.

Eye Massages and Acupressure

Eye massages and acupressure are two techniques that can be used to improve eye health and reduce the risk of myopia. In this book, we will discuss the latest research on the subject and provide practical tips and techniques for incorporating these techniques into your daily routine.

Eye massages can help to relieve eye strain, improve circulation, and reduce the risk of myopia. They can be performed by gently massaging the temples, around the eyes, and along the eyebrows. These massages can be performed several times a day, and should be done in a quiet and dark environment to allow the eyes to rest and relax.

Acupressure is a technique that involves applying pressure to specific points on the body to relieve tension and improve health. For the eyes, there are several acupressure points that can be used to relieve eye strain and improve eye health. These points can be found around the eyes, temples, and eyebrows, and can be stimulated by gently massaging or pressing them.

By incorporating eye massages and acupressure into your daily routine, you can improve your eye health and reduce your risk of myopia. In this book, we will provide guidance and support to help you implement these techniques and achieve your vision improvement goals.

Focus Exercises and Visualization Techniques

Focus exercises and visualization techniques are two approaches that can be used to improve vision and reduce the risk of myopia. In this book, we will discuss the latest research on the subject and provide practical tips and techniques for incorporating these approaches into your daily routine.

Focus exercises are designed to improve visual acuity and strengthen the eye muscles. They can include techniques such as eye tracking, focusing on objects at different distances, and alternating between near and far objects. These exercises can be performed several times a day, and should be done in a well-lit environment to allow the eyes to adjust to different light levels.

Visualization techniques are designed to improve visual acuity and reduce eye strain. They can include techniques such as imagining bright and clear images, visualizing a peaceful and relaxing environment, and focusing on the present moment. These techniques can be performed at any time, and can help to reduce stress and anxiety while improving eye health.

By incorporating focus exercises and visualization techniques into your daily routine, you can improve your vision and reduce your risk of myopia. In this book, we will provide guidance and support to help you implement

these approaches and achieve your vision improvement
goals.

Dynamic Visual Training

Dynamic visual training is a technique that is designed to improve visual acuity and reduce the risk of myopia. It involves performing exercises that challenge the eyes to move and focus in different ways, helping to strengthen the eye muscles and improve visual performance. In this book, we will discuss the latest research on dynamic visual training and provide practical tips and techniques for incorporating this approach into your daily routine.

Dynamic visual training exercises can include tasks such as tracking moving objects, focusing on objects at different distances, and alternating between near and far objects. These exercises can be performed several times a day, and should be done in a well-lit environment to allow the eyes to adjust to different light levels.

Dynamic visual training is a proven and effective way to improve visual acuity and reduce the risk of myopia. In this book, we will provide guidance and support to help you implement this technique and achieve your vision improvement goals. Whether you are looking to improve your overall vision or reduce your risk of nearsightedness, dynamic visual training can be an important part of your vision improvement plan.

Chapter 4. Customizing Your Vision Improvement Plan

Everyone's eyes are unique and what works best for one person may not work as well for another. That's why it's important to customize your vision improvement plan to meet your individual needs and goals.

In this section of the book, we will provide guidance and support to help you create a customized vision improvement plan that works best for you. This may include a combination of lifestyle changes, eye exercises, visualization techniques, and other approaches that have been shown to be effective for improving vision and reducing the risk of myopia. This includes changes to your diet, reducing your screen time, incorporating eye exercises into your daily routine, and more.

By customizing your vision improvement plan, you can maximize your chances of success and achieve the best possible results. The information, guidance, and support you need to take control of your eye health and improve your vision naturally will be provided .

Assessing Your Current Vision Status

Before you can begin to improve your vision, it is important to assess your current vision status. This will help you to determine your baseline and set realistic goals for improvement. In this section of the book, we will discuss how to assess your current vision status and what factors may be contributing to your nearsightedness.

The first step in assessing your vision status is to have a comprehensive eye exam. This should be done by an optometrist or ophthalmologist who can evaluate your eye health and visual acuity. During the exam, they will measure the curvature of your cornea and the length of your eye, and they may use a variety of tests to assess your visual function.

It is also important to keep track of any changes in your vision over time. This can be done by tracking your visual acuity, noting any changes in the quality of your vision, and reporting any symptoms such as eye strain, headaches, or fatigue.

In addition to a comprehensive eye exam, there are other factors that may contribute to your nearsightedness. These can include genetics, excessive screen time, a lack of outdoor light exposure, and more. In this book, we will discuss these factors in more detail and provide guidance on how to address them.

By assessing your current vision status, you can better understand your eye health and set realistic goals for improvement. In this book, we will provide the information and support you need to assess your vision status and take control of your eye health.

Setting Realistic Goals

Once you have assessed your current vision status, the next step is to set realistic goals for improvement. This will help you to focus your efforts and measure your progress over time. In this section of the book, we will discuss how to set realistic goals and what you can expect from your vision improvement plan.

When setting your goals, it is important to consider your current vision status, any underlying health conditions, and the specific factors that may be contributing to your nearsightedness. For example, if you spend a lot of time looking at digital screens, your goal might be to reduce your screen time and incorporate eye exercises into your daily routine.

It is also important to set achievable and realistic goals. For example, if you have a high degree of nearsightedness, it may not be possible to achieve perfect 20/20 vision, but you may be able to significantly improve your visual acuity and reduce the progression of your nearsightedness.

In this book, we will provide guidance on how to set realistic goals and what you can expect from your vision improvement plan. We will also discuss the different vision improvement techniques and approaches that have been shown to be effective for reducing the risk of myopia and improving visual acuity.

By setting realistic goals and following a customized vision improvement plan, you can take control of your eye health and improve your vision naturally. With the information and support provided in this book, you can achieve your best possible vision and reduce the risk of nearsightedness.

Incorporating Techniques and Lifestyle Changes into Your Daily Routine

In order to achieve your goals and improve your vision, it is important to incorporate the techniques and lifestyle changes discussed in this book into your daily routine. This will help you to make lasting changes and establish healthy habits that support your eye health. In this section of the book, we will discuss how to incorporate the techniques and lifestyle changes into your daily routine and what you can expect from the process.

One of the key components of a successful vision improvement plan is consistency. By incorporating the techniques and lifestyle changes into your daily routine, you will be able to establish healthy habits and make lasting changes to your eye health.

The specific techniques and lifestyle changes you choose to incorporate will depend on your individual goals and the specific factors contributing to your nearsightedness. For example, if you spend a lot of time looking at digital screens, you may want to focus on reducing your screen time and incorporating eye exercises into your daily routine. If you have a sedentary lifestyle, you may want to focus on incorporating more physical activity into your day.

In this book, we will provide guidance on how to incorporate the techniques and lifestyle changes into your daily routine, and what you can expect from the process. We will also provide tips and tricks to help you stay motivated and on track with your vision improvement plan.

By incorporating the techniques and lifestyle changes into your daily routine, you can take control of your eye health and achieve your goals for improving your vision. With the information and support provided in this book, you can achieve your best possible vision and reduce the risk of nearsightedness.

Monitoring Progress and Making Adjustments as Needed

In order to achieve your goals and improve your vision, it is important to monitor your progress and make adjustments as needed. This will help you to see the results of your efforts and make any necessary changes to your vision improvement plan. In this section of the book, we will discuss how to monitor your progress and make adjustments as needed.

It is important to track your progress regularly and assess the impact of the techniques and lifestyle changes you have incorporated into your daily routine. This will help you to identify areas where you need to make adjustments and determine what is working well for you.

In this book, we will provide guidance on how to monitor your progress and make adjustments as needed. We will also provide tips on how to track your progress and what to look for when assessing the impact of your vision improvement plan.

If you find that your progress is not what you expected, it may be necessary to make adjustments to your vision improvement plan. This could mean incorporating additional techniques, making changes to your lifestyle, or seeking the support of a healthcare provider.

By monitoring your progress and making adjustments as needed, you can achieve your goals and improve your vision. With the information and support provided in this book, you can achieve your best possible vision and reduce the risk of nearsightedness.

Chapter 5. Maintaining Good Eye Health

Maintaining good eye health is an ongoing process that requires ongoing effort and attention. In this section of the book, we will discuss how to maintain good eye health and keep your vision in top condition.

Once you have achieved your goals for improving your vision, it is important to continue to make eye health a priority. This will help you to maintain the results you have achieved and reduce the risk of nearsightedness in the future.

In this book, we will provide guidance on how to maintain good eye health and keep your vision in top condition. We will discuss the importance of continuing to incorporate the techniques and lifestyle changes discussed in this book into your daily routine, as well as other strategies for maintaining good eye health.

It is also important to have regular eye exams and eye health screenings, even if your vision has improved. This will help you to detect any changes in your eye health and address any potential problems early.

By maintaining good eye health and keeping your vision in top condition, you can enjoy clear, healthy vision for years to come. With the information and support provided in this book, you can achieve and maintain your best possible vision.

The Importance of Regular Eye Exams

Regular eye exams are an essential part of maintaining good eye health and keeping your vision in top condition. In this section of the book, we will discuss the importance of regular eye exams and why they are essential for maintaining good eye health.

Eye exams can help to detect and prevent a wide range of eye health problems, including nearsightedness, farsightedness, astigmatism, and more. They can also help to detect other health conditions, such as high blood pressure, diabetes, and other conditions that can affect eye health.

During an eye exam, your eye doctor will examine your eyes and test your vision. They will also evaluate your overall eye health, including your eye muscles, eye movement, and other key indicators. Based on this evaluation, they will be able to make recommendations for maintaining good eye health and improving your vision.

In this book, we will discuss the importance of regular eye exams and provide tips on how to find a qualified eye doctor. We will also discuss the different types of eye exams, including comprehensive eye exams, contact lens exams, and other types of exams.

By having regular eye exams, you can ensure that your
eye health is in top condition and detect any potential
problems early. With the information and support
provided in this book, you can achieve and maintain
your best possible vision.

Tips for Protecting Your Eyes from Harm

Myopia, also known as nearsightedness, is a common eye condition that affects millions of people worldwide. This condition makes it difficult to see objects in the distance and can be corrected with glasses or contact lenses. However, it's also important to protect your eyes from further damage to maintain good eye health and reduce the risk of developing more serious conditions in the future. Here are some tips to help protect your eyes and prevent myopia from getting worse:

Wear protective eyewear: If you engage in activities that may harm your eyes, such as playing sports or working with power tools, make sure to wear protective eyewear to shield your eyes from injury.

Limit screen time: Spending too much time looking at digital screens can put a strain on your eyes and contribute to myopia progression. Try to take breaks every 20-30 minutes and look away from the screen to reduce eye strain.

Maintain good lighting: Poor lighting can strain your eyes, especially when reading or working on the computer. Make sure the lighting in your work or study environment is bright and evenly distributed to reduce eye strain.

Practice good posture: Good posture can reduce the strain on your eyes, especially when reading or working on the computer. Make sure your computer screen is at eye level, and sit up straight to reduce neck and back pain.

Get regular eye exams: Regular eye exams are important for monitoring the progression of myopia and detecting other eye conditions. Your eye doctor can also advise you on the best corrective measures, such as glasses or contact lenses, to help you see clearly.

Wear sunglasses: Ultraviolet (UV) rays from the sun can harm your eyes and increase the risk of developing cataracts and other eye conditions. Make sure to wear sunglasses that offer UV protection whenever you're outdoors.

Maintain a healthy diet: A healthy diet that includes plenty of fruits, vegetables, and essential nutrients can help maintain good eye health and reduce the risk of developing eye conditions, such as myopia.

By following these tips, you can help protect your eyes from further harm and maintain good eye health. If you have any concerns about your eye health, make sure to see an eye doctor for a comprehensive eye exam.

Continuing Your Vision Improvement Journey

Maintaining good eye health and improving your vision is a lifelong journey, and it's important to take the necessary steps to keep your eyes healthy and strong. Here are some tips to help you continue your vision improvement journey:

Stay active: Regular physical activity is important for maintaining good overall health, including eye health. Engage in activities such as walking, jogging, cycling, or swimming to keep your body and eyes in good condition.

Get enough sleep: Adequate sleep is essential for eye health and overall health. Aim for at least 7-8 hours of sleep each night to help your eyes and body regenerate and recover.

Quit smoking: Smoking has been linked to a number of eye conditions, including age-related macular degeneration and cataracts. Quitting smoking can help reduce the risk of developing these conditions and improve your overall eye health.

Wear protective eyewear: If you engage in activities that may harm your eyes, such as playing sports or working with power tools, make sure to wear protective eyewear to shield your eyes from injury.

Eat a healthy diet: A healthy diet that includes plenty of fruits, vegetables, and essential nutrients can help maintain good eye health and reduce the risk of developing eye conditions.

Manage stress: Chronic stress can contribute to eye problems and overall health issues. Make time for activities that help you relax and manage stress, such as yoga, meditation, or simply taking a walk.

Get regular eye exams: Regular eye exams are important for monitoring your eye health and detecting any changes or conditions that may require treatment. Your eye doctor can also advise you on the best corrective measures, such as glasses or contact lenses, to help you see clearly.

By following these tips, you can continue your vision improvement journey and maintain good eye health. Remember, taking care of your eyes is a lifelong commitment, so make sure to prioritize your eye health and seek help from an eye doctor if you have any concerns.

Food that are beneficial to Improving eye health

What you eat can have a significant impact on your eye health and vision. Incorporating certain foods into your diet can help improve your eye health and reduce the risk of developing eye conditions. Here are some foods that are beneficial for improving eye health:

Leafy greens: Foods like spinach, kale, and collard greens are high in vitamins A, C, and E, as well as lutein and zeaxanthin, two important nutrients for eye health.

Fish: Fish such as salmon, mackerel, and sardines are rich in omega-3 fatty acids, which have been shown to help reduce the risk of age-related macular degeneration and other eye conditions.

Nuts and seeds: Nuts and seeds, such as almonds, walnuts, and chia seeds, are high in vitamins and minerals, such as vitamin E and zinc, that are important for eye health.

Eggs: Eggs are a great source of lutein and zeaxanthin, as well as vitamins A and D, which are important for maintaining good eye health.

Citrus fruits: Citrus fruits, such as oranges, lemons, and limes, are high in vitamin C, which helps protect the eyes from damage caused by free radicals.

Berries: Berries, such as blueberries, raspberries, and blackberries, are high in antioxidants that help protect the eyes from oxidative stress and damage.

Whole grains: Whole grains, such as brown rice and whole wheat, are high in vitamins and minerals, such as vitamin B and magnesium, that are important for maintaining good eye health.

Incorporating these foods into your diet can help improve your eye health and reduce the risk of developing eye conditions. However, it's important to remember that a balanced diet and regular exercise are also essential for maintaining good overall health, including eye health. If you have any concerns about your eye health, make sure to see an eye doctor for a comprehensive eye exam.

Chapter 6. Conclusion

In conclusion, taking care of your eyes and maintaining good eye health is essential for ensuring clear vision and reducing the risk of developing eye conditions. Simple steps, such as eating a healthy diet, getting enough sleep, and wearing protective eyewear, can help improve your eye health and protect your vision. Regular eye exams are also important for monitoring your eye health and detecting any changes or conditions that may require treatment.

By following these tips and incorporating eye-healthy habits into your daily routine, you can help maintain good eye health and continue to enjoy clear vision for years to come. If you have any concerns about your eye health, make sure to see an eye doctor for a comprehensive eye exam and advice on the best course of action. Your eyes are an important part of your overall health, so make sure to prioritize your eye health and take the necessary steps to protect your vision.

The Benefits of Improving Your Vision Naturally

Improving your vision naturally is a safe, effective way to maintain good eye health and protect your vision. There are several benefits to improving your vision naturally, including:

Avoiding harmful chemicals and side effects: Many conventional treatments for eye conditions, such as surgery and prescription eye drops, can cause side effects and potentially harmful chemicals. Improving your vision naturally, on the other hand, allows you to avoid these risks and improve your eye health in a safe, natural way.

Reducing the risk of eye conditions: Incorporating healthy habits, such as eating a balanced diet, getting enough sleep, and engaging in regular physical activity, into your routine can help reduce the risk of developing eye conditions, such as cataracts and age-related macular degeneration.

Improving overall health: Improving your vision naturally also has the added benefit of improving your overall health. A healthy lifestyle, including a balanced diet, regular exercise, and stress management, can have a positive impact on your overall well-being and reduce the risk of developing other health problems.

Cost savings: Conventional treatments for eye conditions, such as surgery and prescription eye drops, can be expensive. Improving your vision naturally, on the other hand, often requires only small lifestyle changes, which can save you money and improve your eye health at the same time.

Empowerment: Improving your vision naturally empowers you to take control of your eye health and make positive changes that can improve your vision and overall well-being.

Incorporating healthy habits into your daily routine and making small lifestyle changes can have a big impact on your eye health and vision. If you have any concerns about your eye health, make sure to see an eye doctor for a comprehensive eye exam and advice on the best course of action. Improving your vision naturally is a safe, effective way to maintain good eye health and protect your vision for years to come.

Final Thoughts and Encouragement

Taking care of your eye health is essential for maintaining good vision and reducing the risk of developing eye conditions. Improving your vision naturally, by incorporating healthy habits and making small lifestyle changes, is a safe, effective way to do so.

It's important to remember that taking care of your eye health is a journey, not a destination. Making small, gradual changes can have a big impact over time and help you maintain good eye health for years to come. Whether you're looking to improve your vision, reduce the risk of eye conditions, or simply prioritize your health, there are many ways to improve your eye health naturally.

So take the first step today, and make eye health a priority in your life. Whether it's eating a healthy diet, getting enough sleep, or wearing protective eyewear, every little bit helps. And remember, if you have any concerns about your eye health, make sure to see an eye doctor for a comprehensive eye exam and advice on the best course of action.

Here's to your continued good eye health and clear vision!

Remember, it's important to prioritize your eye health and take the necessary steps to protect your vision. By using these resources and incorporating healthy habits into your daily routine, you can continue your vision improvement journey and maintain good eye health for years to come.